DIABETES DURING PREGNANCY

(Gravid Diabetes)

Causes, Risk Factors, Symptoms, Consequences, And Treatment Of **Gravid** Diabetes.

By

Daphne E. Howard

TABLE OF CONTENT

INTRODUCTION

Diabetes is a habitual, metabolic condition marked by increased situations of blood glucose(or blood sugar), which leads over time to disastrous damage to the heart, blood vessels, eyes, feathers, and jitters. The most common is type 2 diabetes, substantially in grown-ups, which arises when the body becomes resistant to insulin or does not produce enough insulin. In the once three decades, the frequency of type 2 diabetes has risen fleetly in countries of all income situations. Type 1 diabetes, historically known as juvenile diabetes or insulin-dependent diabetes, is a habitual illness in which the pancreas produces little or no insulin by itself. For those living with diabetes, access to affordable drugs, particularly insulin, is vital to their survival. There's an encyclopedically honored ideal to halt the rise in diabetes and rotundity by 2025. About 422 million people worldwide have diabetes, the maturity abiding in low- and middle-income countries and 1.5 million deaths are directly related to diabetes each time. Both the number of cases and the frequency of diabetes have been continuously growing over the once many decades. Still, you should go on to have a healthy baby, if you become pregnant and have diabetes. But there are some possible issues you should be apprehensive of. The information in this book applies to you if you were diagnosed with type 1 or type 2 diabetes before you got pregnant. It covers gravid diabetes, which is high blood sugar that occurs during gestation and it typically goes down after the baby is born.

CHAPTER 1
DIABETICS AND GESTATION

Gravid (GESTATIONAL) diabetes is characterized by elevated situations of glucose (blood sugar) that manifest themselves throughout gestation and generally dwindle after the delivery of the baby. The alternate or third trimester of gestation is the most usual time for it to be done; still, it can be done at any stage of gestation. Your body is unfit to produce enough insulin, which is a hormone that helps manage blood sugar situations, to satisfy your increased conditions during gestation. This condition is known as gravid diabetes. Both during gestation and after delivery, you and your future child may witness complications as a result of gravid diabetes. Still, if the illness is linked at an early stage and effectively handled, the hazards can be eased.

WHAT IT MEANS FOR YOU

Still, you may be at an increased threat of having if you have diabetes of either type 1 or type 2.

• A huge baby, which raises the liability of having a delicate birth, taking a convinced labor fashion, or having a cesarean section to deliver the baby. A loss of gestation People who have diabetes, regardless of whether or not they're pregnant, are at threat of developing complications with their feathers and eyes, which are appertained to as diabetic nephropathy and diabetic retinopathy, independently. Some people with type 1 diabetes can develop diabetic ketoacidosis when dangerous motes called ketones make up in the blood. Gestation can increase your threat of acquiring some diseases or make living bone Worse.

WHAT IT MEANS FOR YOUR BABY

Still, your baby may be at advanced risk if you have type 1 or type 2 diabetes.

• having health problems shortly after delivery, similar to heart and breathing problems, and demanding sanitarium care

• developing fat or diabetes later in life There is also a slightly larger peril of your sprat being born with birth problems, including heart and nervous system abnormalities, or being stillborn or dying soon after birth. Still, controlling your diabetes rightly ahead and during gestation will help to lessen these pitfalls.

CHAPTER 2
REDUCING THE PITFALLS OF GRAVID DIABETES

The stylish system to reduce the troubles for you and your baby is to ensure your diabetes is well controlled before you become pregnant. So, immaculately, a gestation should be planned. Before you start trying for a baby, ask your GP or diabetes specialist (dialectologist) for guidance. You should be referred to a diabetic pre-conception clinic for help. It would help if you were offered a blood test, called an HbA1c test, every month. This measures the position of glucose in your blood. It's optimal if the position is no higher than 6.5 before you get pregnant. If you cannot bring your position below 6.5, attempt to get it as close as possible to lessen the threat of issues for you and your baby. Still, your care team should explosively encourage you not to try for a baby until it has been reduced. If your blood glucose level is above 10. You should continue using contraceptives until you bring your blood glucose under control. A GP or diabetic specialist can advise you on how to achieve this. Still, you should be given testing strips and an examiner to estimate your blood ketone levels if you have type 1 diabetes. To screen for diabetic ketoacidosis, you should use them if your blood glucose levels are high, if you're ill, or if you have diarrhea. If you have diabetes and are trying to conceive, you should take 5 milligrams (mg) of folic acid per day (or until you are 12 weeks pregnant). A croaker.

You will have to define this because you cannot get 5 mg tablets from a drugstore or supermarket without a tradition. Taking folic acid can prevent your baby from developing birth abnormalities, similar to spina bifida.

WHO IS AT RISK FOR GRAVID DIABETES?

Any woman can develop gravid diabetes during gestation; still, you are at an elevated threat if:

• You're over 40;

• Your body mass index (BMI) is above 30;

• You preliminary had a baby who counted 4.5 kg (10 lb.) or further at birth;

• You had gravid diabetes in a former gestation;

• One of your parents or siblings has diabetes;

• You're of South Asian, black, African-Caribbean, or Middle Eastern origin (indeed if you were born in the UK);

• You have had a gastric bypass or other weight-loss surgery;

SYMPTOMS OF GRAVID DIABETES.

Gravid diabetes doesn't typically produce any symptoms. Most cases are only set up when your blood sugar levels are measured during the webbing for gravid diabetes. Some women may suffer symptoms if their blood sugar levels are too high (hyperglycemia), such as increased thirst, demanding to pee more frequently than usual, a dry mouth, frazzle, blurred sight, or genital itching or thrush. Some of these symptoms are common throughout gestation and aren't inescapably a sign of gravid diabetes. Speak to your midwife or croaker

If you are upset about any symptoms you are passing.

CHAPTER 3
HOW GRAVID DIABETES MIGHT AFFECT YOUR PREGNANCY.

Utmost women with gravid diabetes have else normal gravidity with healthy kiddies. Still, gravid diabetes can beget issues similar to

• Your baby is developing larger than usual- this may lead to complications during the delivery and raises the probability of having artificial labor or a cesarean section.

• Polyhydramnios – too important amniotic fluid (the fluid that surrounds the baby) in the womb, which can induce unseasonable labor or complications at delivery

• Unseasonable delivery – giving birth before the 37th week of gestation

•Pre-eclampsia – a complaint that causes high blood pressure during gestation and can lead to gestation difficulties if not managed.

• Your baby suffering low blood sugar or yellowing of the skin and eyes (hostility) after he or she's delivered, which may bear treatment in a sanitarium

• the loss of your baby(birth)- though this is unusual
Having gravid diabetes also implies you are at an elevated threat of getting type 2 diabetes in the future.

WEBBING OR SCREENING FOR GRAVID DIABETES

During your first prenatal scan(occasionally called a booking appointment) at around weeks 8 to 12 of your gestation, your midwife or croaker will ask you certain questions to establish whether you are at an increased threat of gravid diabetes. If you have 1 or further threat factors for gravid diabetes you should be offered a webbing test. The webbing test is nominated as an oral glucose forbearance test (OGTT), which takes around 2 hours. It entails having a blood test in the morning when you haven't had any food or drink for 8 to 10 hours (though you can typically belt water, but check with the sanitarium if you are doubtful). You are also handed a glucose drink. After resting for 2 hours, another blood sample is collected to determine how your body is responding to the glucose. The OGTT is done when you are between 24 and 28 weeks pregnant. However, you will be offered an OGTT before your gestation, incontinently after your booking discussion, if you've had gravid diabetes ahead.

DIABETIC EYE WEBBING OR SCREENING IN GESTATION

You'll be offered regular diabetic eye webbing during your gestation. This is to look for symptoms of diabetic eye complaint (diabetic retinopathy) Webbing is especially important when you're pregnant because the threat of significant eye issues is advanced in gestation. Diabetic retinopathy is treatable, especially if it's discovered beforehand. Still, you should advise the clinician looking after your diabetes treatment during gestation, if you conclude not to have regular webbing tests.

CHAPTER 4
TREATMENTS FOR GRAVID DIABETES

Still, the odds of having issues with your gestation can be minimized by regulating your blood sugar situation, if you have gravid diabetes. You will be given a blood sugar testing tackle so you can cover the impact of treatment. Blood sugar situations may be dropped by modifying your diet and getting more active if you can. Gentle exercises similar to walking, swimming, and

antenatal
yoga can help lower blood sugar. But tell your midwife
or croaker
before bearing an exertion you haven't done ahead.
Still, if these variations do not drop your blood sugar
situation enough, you'll need to take drugs as well. This
may be tablets or insulin injections. You will also be
more completely checked during your gestation and
birth to look for any implicit complications. Still, it's
ideal to deliver birth before 41 weeks, if you have
gravid diabetes. Induction of labor or a cesarean section
may be considered if labor doesn't start naturally by this
time. Before birth may be considered if there are
enterprises about your or your baby's health or if your
blood sugar situation hasn't been effectively controlled.
Your diabetes remedy in gestation your croakers
may propose modifying your treatment routine during
gestation. Still, you will typically be advised to switch
to insulin injections, either with or without a medicine
called metformin, if you generally take tablets to
control your diabetes. Still, you may need to switch to a
new type of insulin, if you formerly need insulin
injections to control your diabetes. Still, similar to high
blood pressure, they may have to be altered, if you take
medicines for problems connected to your diabetes. It's
vitally important to attend to any movables planned for

you so that your care platoon can cover your status and reply to any changes that could impact your or your baby's health. You'll need to cover your blood glucose situations more regularly throughout gestation, especially since nausea and puking in gestation (known as "morning sickness", although it can be at any time of the day) might alter them. Your GP or midwife will be suitable to advise you on this. Keeping your blood glucose situations low may mean you suffer lower blood-sugar (hypoglycemic) attacks (" hypos"). These are inoffensive for your baby, but you and your mate need to know how to manage with them. Talk to your croaker or diabetes specialist.

LONG-TERM EFFECT OF GRAVID DIABETES

Generally goes down after birth. But women who've had it are more prone to develop

• Gravid diabetes again in unborn gravidity

• Type 2 diabetes – a lifelong type of diabetes you should get a blood test to check for diabetes 6 to 13 weeks after giving birth, and formerly per time after that if the result is normal. See your GP if you witness signs of high blood sugar, similar to increased thirst, demanding to pee more frequently than normal, and a dry mouth- don't stay until you're coming test. You should get the tests indeed if you feel fine, as numerous people with diabetes don't have any symptoms. You will also be told about the effects you can do to lower your chance of acquiring diabetes, similar to keeping a healthy weight, eating a balanced diet, and exercising regularly. Some studies have revealed that babies of mothers who had gravid diabetes may be more prone to develop diabetes or become fat later in life.

CHAPTER 5
SAFETY WAYS FOR GRAVID DIABETES DURING PREGNANCY

Still, the chances of having problems with the gestation can be reduced by controlling your blood sugar (glucose) situations, if you have gravid diabetes. You will also need to be more nearly covered during gestation and labor to check if treatment is working and for any problems.

CHECKING YOUR BLOOD SUGAR POSITION

You will be given a testing tackle that you can use to check your blood sugar (glucose) position. This involves using a cutlet-poking device and putting a drop of blood on a testing strip. You will be advised

• How to test your blood sugar position rightly

• When and how frequently to test your blood sugar – you will generally be advised to test before breakfast and 1 hour after each mess

• What position you should be aiming for – this will be a dimension given in mill moles of glucose per liter of blood (mmol/ l)

• How to partake your blood sugar situations with your care platoon, to help you get the right advice and treatment still, your care platoon might offer you a nonstop glucose examiner (CGM), if you take insulin and have problems with low blood sugar (hypoglycemia) or your blood sugar isn't stable. This is a small detector you wear on your skin that sends data wirelessly to a receiver or a mobile phone, so you can see your blood sugar position at any time.

A HEALTHY DIET

Making changes to your diet can help control your blood sugar situation. You should be appertained to a dietitian, who can give you advice about your diet and how to plan healthy reflection. You may be advised to

• eat regularly – generally three refection a day – and avoid skipping refection

• eat stiff and low glycemic indicator(GI) foods that release sugar sluggishly – similar to whole-wheat pasta, brown rice, granary chuck
, all-bran cereals, beats, sap, lentils, muesli and plain porridge

• eat a plenitude of fruit and vegetables – end for at least FIVE PORTION A DAY

• avoid sticky foods – you don't need a fully sugar-free diet, but exchange snacks similar as galettes and biscuits for healthier druthers
similar to fruit, nuts, and seeds

• avoid sticky drinks – diet or sugar-free drinks are better than sticky performances. Fruit authorities and smoothies can also be high in sugar, and so can some" no more sugar" drinks, so check the nutrition marker or ask your healthcare platoon

• eat spare sources of protein, similar to fish It's also important to be apprehensive of foods to avoid during gestation, similar to certain types of fish and rubbish.

Exercise Physical exertion lowers your blood glucose position, so regular exercise can be an effective way to manage gravid diabetes. You will be advised about safe ways to exercise during gestation. A common recommendation is to aim for at least 150 twinkles (2 hours and 30 twinkles) of moderate-intensity exertion a week, plus strength exercises on 2 or further days a week.

MEDICINE

You may be given a drug if your blood sugar situation is still not stable 1 to 2 weeks after changing your diet and exercising regularly, or if your blood sugar position is veritably high when you are first diagnosed. This may be tablets – generally metformin – or insulin injections. Your blood sugar situation can increase as your gestation progresses, so indeed if they ameliorate at first, you may need to take drugs later in gestation. You can generally stop taking these drugs after you give birth.

TABLETS

Metformin is taken as a tablet up to 3 times a day, generally with or after refections. Side effects of metformin can include

• feeling sick

• being sick

• Stomach cramps

• Diarrhea

• Loss of appetite

Sometimes a different tablet called glibenclamide may be specified.

INSULIN

Insulin may be recommended if

• You cannot take metformin or it causes side goods

• Metformin doesn't lower your blood sugar situations enough

• You have veritably high blood sugar

• Your baby is veritably large or you have too important fluid in your womb (polyhydramnios) you fit insulin using an insulin pen. This is a device that helps you fit safely and take the right cure. Using an insulin pen doesn't generally hurt. The needles are veritably small, as you only fit a small quantum just under your skin. You will be shown where to fit and how to use your pen. Depending on the type of insulin you are specified, you may need to take it before refections, at bedtime, or on waking. You'll be told how important insulin is to take. Blood sugar situations generally increase as gestation progresses, so your insulin cure may need to be increased over time. Insulin can cause your blood sugar to fall too low (hypoglycemia). Symptoms of low blood sugar include feeling shaky, sweaty, or empty, turning paler than usual, or chancing it delicately to concentrate. Still, test your blood sugar, and treat it straight down if it's low, if this happens. You will be given information about hypoglycemia if you are specified insulin.

MONITORING YOUR PREGNANCY DURING GESTATION

Gravid diabetes can increase the threat of your baby developing problems, similar to growing larger than usual. Because of this, you will be offered redundant prenatal movables so your baby can be covered. Movables you should be offered include

• An ultrasound checkup at around week 18 to 20 of your gestation to check your baby for abnormalities

• Ultrasound reviews at weeks 28, 32, and 36 – to cover your baby's growth and the quantum of amniotic fluid, plus regular checks from week 38 onwards

Giving birth

The ideal time to give birth if you have gravid diabetes is generally around weeks 38 to 40. Still, you may be suitable to stay for labor to start naturally, if your blood sugar is within normal situations and there are no enterprises about your or your baby's health. Still, you will generally be offered induction of labor or a cesarean section if you haven't given birth by 40 weeks and 6 days. Before delivery may be recommended if there are enterprises about your or your baby's health, or if your blood sugar situation hasn't been well controlled. You should give birth at a sanitarium where specially trained healthcare professionals are available to give applicable care for your baby. When you go into the sanitarium to give birth, take your blood sugar testing tackle with you, plus any drugs you are taking. Generally, you should keep testing your blood sugar and taking your drugs until you are in established labor or you are told to stop eating before a cesarean section. During labor and delivery, your blood sugar will be covered and kept under control. You may need to have insulin given to you through a drip, to control your blood sugar situations.

CHAPTER 6
LABOR AND BIRTH

Still, it's explosively suggested that you give birth in a sanitarium with the care of an adviser-led motherliness platoon if you have diabetes. Your croakers May consider having your labor started beforehand (convinced). This is because there may be an increased threat of difficulties for you or your baby if your gestation drags on for too long. Still, your croakers might bandy your options for the delivery and may propose an optional cesarean section, if your baby is larger than anticipated. Your blood glucose should be covered every hour during labor and birth. You may be given a drip in your arm with insulin and glucose if there are difficulties.

AFTER THE BIRTH

Feed your child as soon as possible after the delivery (within 30 twinkles) to help keep their blood glucose in a safe position. Your child will admit a heel burrow blood test (or invigorated blood spot test) many hours after they are born to check if their blood glucose position is too low. Still, or they are passing issues feeding, they may need redundant care, if your baby's blood glucose cannot be managed at a safe position. Your child may need to be fed through a tube or given a drip to raise their blood glucose. After your gestation, you shouldn't bear as important insulin to control your blood glucose. You should be able to drop your insulin to your pre-pregnancy cure or return to the tablets you were taking before you became pregnant. Talk to your croaker about this. You should be offered a test to assess your blood glucose situation before you leave home and during your 6-week postnatal check, you should also be given information about nutrition and exertion.

PLANNING UNBORN GRAVIDITY (PREGNANCY)

Still, make sure you get checked for diabetes, if you've had gravid diabetes ahead and you are hoping to get pregnant. Your GP can arrange this. Still, you should appertain to a diabetes-conception clinic for support to ensure your condition is adequately controlled before you get pregnant if you do have diabetes. Still, talk to your GP and tell them you endured gravid diabetes in your previous gestation if you have an unexpected gestation. Still, you will be offered webbing before gestation (incontinently after your first midwife appointment) and another test at 24 to 28 weeks if the first test is normal, if tests show you don't have diabetes. Alternatively, your midwife or croaker may propose you cover your blood sugar situations yourself using a cutlet-poking device in the same way as you did during your previous gravid diabetes.

CONCLUSION

Diabetes that isn't well controlled causes the baby's blood sugar to be high. The baby is "overfed" and grows extra-large. Besides causing discomfort to the woman during the last many months of pregnancy, an extra-large baby can lead to problems during delivery for both the mother and the baby, always go for a Glucose wirework check for gravid diabetes. It's important to diagnose the condition because it can beget health problems in an invigorated baby, especially if it's not treated. Most people who have gravid diabetes give birth to healthy babies, especially when they keep their blood sugar under control, eat a healthy diet, get regular, moderate physical exertion, and gain the right quantum of weight. But if left undressed, gravid diabetes can beget serious health problems for you and your baby. As well as the below, nonstop high blood sugar situations can also lead to convinced labor.